AUTOIMMUNE ENCEPHALITIS NUTRITION

How To Heal, Understand Nutrient Essentials, Meal Planning, Brain Health Strategies, Lifestyle Tips, And Delicious Recipes For Enhanced Well-Being

Dr. Holmgren Alfred

The book "Autoimmune Encephalitis Nutrition: Expert Guidance" offers a comprehensive exploration into the intricate relationship between nutrition and the management of autoimmune encephalitis, a condition that affects the brain and requires careful attention to diet and lifestyle.

By delving into the nuances of this autoimmune disorder, the book sheds light on the origins, symptoms, and diagnosis, empowering readers with a deeper understanding of their condition.

With expert-backed advice, readers gain valuable knowledge on crafting a nutrient-rich diet plan tailored to their unique health requirements, from proteins and amino acids to vitamins and minerals. Navigating the labyrinth of autoimmune encephalitis requires a nuanced approach, and this book serves as a trusted guide, offering insights into the specific nutritional needs of individuals with this condition.

Furthermore, "Autoimmune Encephalitis Nutrition: Expert Guidance" emphasizes the crucial connection between gut health and brain function, revealing the profound impact of dietary choices on cognitive well-being.

Through meticulous exploration of lifestyle factors, including stress management techniques and exercise recommendations, the book empowers readers to cultivate a holistic approach to autoimmune encephalitis management, fostering resilience and vitality.

Recognizing the challenges inherent in adopting dietary changes, the book offers practical strategies for addressing food sensitivities, navigating medication interactions, and managing the social and emotional aspects of lifestyle changes.

With a treasure trove of recipes and meal ideas, readers are equipped to embark on a culinary journey that not only nurtures the body but also delights the palate.

Furthermore, "Autoimmune Encephalitis Nutrition: Expert Guidance" extends beyond the confines of its pages, providing readers with a roadmap to further resources and support networks.

The book serves as a beacon of support for individuals seeking to reclaim their health and vitality in the face of autoimmune encephalitis.

Copyright © Holmgren Alfred 2024.

All rights reserved.

This publication may not be reproduced, distributed, or transmitted in any form or by any means, including photocopying, recording, or other electronic or mechanical methods, without the publisher's written permission, except for brief quotations in critical reviews and other copyright-permitted non-commercial uses. Contact publisher Information for permissions.

This book is fictitious. Authors create names, people, places, and events.

Any resemblance to real events, places, or people—living or dead—is coincidental.

Disclaimer

This book, "Autoimmune Encephalitis Nutrition: With Expert Guidance," is intended to provide general information and guidance on the topic of autoimmune encephalitis and nutrition.

The information contained within this book is based on research, expert opinions, and personal experiences, and is intended to be educational and informative.

It is important to note that I, the author, do not endorse any individual, product, website, organization, or other entity mentioned or referenced in this book; any mention of such entities is solely for informational purposes and does not constitute an endorsement or recommendation.

Readers are advised to use their discretion and consult with qualified healthcare professionals before making any decisions or taking any actions based on the information provided in this book, as each person's health and dietary needs are unique, and what works for one person may not work for another.

Furthermore, while every effort has been made to ensure the accuracy and reliability of the information presented in this book, I make no express or implied representations or warranties about the completeness, accuracy, reliability, suitability, or availability of the content contained herein. As a result, any reliance you place on such information is strictly at your own risk.

In no event shall I, as the author, be liable for any loss or harm, including but not limited to indirect or consequential loss or damage, or any loss or damage whatsoever originating from loss of data or profits deriving from, or in connection with, the use of this book.

By reading this book, you accept and agree to the terms of this disclaimer; if you do not agree with these terms, do not use or depend on the information included in this book.

CHAPTER 1
UNDERSTANDING AUTOIMMUNE ESOPHAGITIS

Autoimmune encephalitis is a rare and potentially serious condition characterized by inflammation of the brain caused by the immune system mistakenly attacking healthy brain cells. In this disorder, antibodies, which are typically produced by the immune system to fight off infections, instead target proteins within or associated with neurons in the brain. This autoimmune response causes a variety of neurological symptoms and can significantly impact cognitive function and behavior.

Herpes simplex virus (HSV), Epstein-Barr virus (EBV), and cytomegalovirus (CMV) have all been linked to autoimmune encephalitis, though the exact mechanisms by which this occurs are not fully understood.

In some cases, autoimmune encephalitis develops spontaneously without a known cause, while in others, it is linked to specific infections, tumors, or other autoimmune disorders.

Autoimmune encephalitis can cause a wide range of neurological symptoms, including seizures, movement disorders, and autonomic dysfunction, as well as cognitive dysfunction like memory loss, confusion, and difficulty concentrating, and psychiatric symptoms like hallucinations, paranoia, and mood disturbances. Diagnosing autoimmune encephalitis can be

The first line of treatment for autoimmune encephalitis is immunotherapy, which may include corticosteroids to reduce inflammation, intravenous immunoglobulin

(IVIG) to modulate the immune system, or plasmapheresis to remove circulating antibodies from the bloodstream. The goal of the treatment is to suppress the abnormal immune response, reduce inflammation in the brain, and effectively manage symptoms. If the first line of treatment is ineffective or the symptoms persist,

CHAPTER 2

THE ROLE OF NUTRITION IN AUTOIMMUNE ESOPHAGITIS

Autoimmune encephalitis is a complex neurological disorder characterized by inflammation of the brain due to an autoimmune response, in which the body's immune system mistakenly attacks healthy brain tissue. While medical interventions such as immunotherapy and corticosteroids are commonly used to manage symptoms and reduce inflammation, the role of nutrition in the management and treatment of autoimmune encephalitis is increasingly recognized.

How Nutrition Affects Autoimmune Conditions:

Nutrition plays a fundamental role in modulating the immune system's function and maintaining its balance.

Certain dietary factors can either exacerbate or alleviate autoimmune conditions like encephalitis. For instance, a diet rich in processed foods, refined sugars, and unhealthy fats can promote inflammation and contribute to immune dysregulation, potentially worsening symptoms of autoimmune encephalitis.

Conversely, a nutrient-dense diet composed of whole foods, including fruits, vegetables, lean proteins, healthy fats, and complex carbohydrates, provides essential nutrients and antioxidants that support immune function and reduce inflammation.

Moreover, specific nutrients such as omega-3 fatty acids, vitamin D, antioxidants, and certain amino acids have been shown to modulate immune responses and attenuate autoimmune reactions, thereby offering potential therapeutic benefits in managing autoimmune encephalitis.

Thus, adopting a balanced and nutrient-rich diet tailored to individual needs is crucial for optimizing immune function and mitigating the severity of autoimmune encephalitis symptoms.

Specific nutritional requirements in autoimmune encephalitis:

Individuals with autoimmune encephalitis may have unique nutritional needs due to the underlying inflammatory processes, neurological dysfunction, and potential side effects of medications used in treatment. Adequate intake of nutrients essential for brain health and immune function is particularly important in managing autoimmune encephalitis. For example, omega-3 fatty acids found in fatty fish, flaxseeds, and walnuts have anti-inflammatory properties and may help reduce neuroinflammation associated with autoimmune encephalitis. Likewise, vitamin D plays a critical role in immune regulation and neuroprotection, and deficiency has been linked to increased autoimmune activity and neurological symptoms. Therefore, ensuring sufficient intake of vitamin D through diet, sunlight exposure, or supplementation may be beneficial for individuals with autoimmune encephalitis. Additionally, antioxidants such as vitamin C, vitamin E, and selenium help neutralize free radicals and reduce oxidative stress, which can exacerbate inflammation and neuronal damage in autoimmune encephalitis. Incorporating antioxidant-rich foods like berries, citrus fruits, nuts, and seeds into the diet can support brain health and enhance resilience against autoimmune-related damage.

Emerging research has highlighted the intricate relationship between the gut and the brain, known as the gut-brain axis, which plays a crucial role in immune regulation, inflammation, and neurological function. Disruptions in the gut microbiota composition, known as dysbiosis, have been implicated in the pathogenesis of autoimmune conditions, including encephalitis. The gut microbiota, comprised of trillions of microorganisms, interacts with the immune system and influences systemic inflammation and autoimmune responses. Imbalances in gut microbial diversity and integrity can lead to increased intestinal permeability (leaky gut), allowing the translocation of microbial products and toxins into the systemic circulation, triggering immune activation and neuroinflammation.

Moreover, the gut microbiota produces various metabolites, including short-chain fatty acids (SCFAs) and neurotransmitters, which can modulate immune function, neuronal signaling, and behavior.

Thus, interventions aimed at restoring gut microbial balance, such as probiotics, prebiotics, dietary fiber, and fermented foods, may have therapeutic potential in autoimmune encephalitis by reducing inflammation, enhancing immune tolerance, and supporting neurological function via the gut-brain axis.

Understanding and targeting the gut-brain connection through dietary interventions offer promising avenues for the management and treatment of autoimmune encephalitis, emphasizing the importance of personalized nutrition approaches in optimizing health outcomes for affected individuals.

nutrition plays a critical role in the management and treatment of autoimmune encephalitis by modulating immune function, reducing inflammation, supporting brain health, and restoring gut microbial balance. Adopting a balanced and nutrient-rich diet tailored to individual needs, along with targeted interventions to address specific nutritional deficiencies and promote gut health, can complement conventional therapies and enhance resilience against autoimmunity.

CHAPTER 3
ESSENTIAL NUTRIENTS FOR AUTOIMMUNE ENCEPHALITIS MANAGEMENT

Proteins and Amino Acids: Proteins and amino acids play a crucial role in managing autoimmune encephalitis by supporting various bodily functions, including immune system regulation and tissue repair. Amino acids are the building blocks of proteins, and they are essential for the synthesis of neurotransmitters, which are vital for proper brain function. In autoimmune encephalitis, where the immune system mistakenly attacks brain cells, adequate protein intake becomes imperative for supporting the repair and regeneration of damaged neural tissues. Furthermore, certain amino acids such as glutamine and glycine have been shown to possess neuroprotective properties, helping to mitigate inflammation and oxidative stress in the brain.

Dietary sources rich in protein and amino acids include lean meats, poultry, fish, eggs, dairy products, legumes, nuts, and seeds. Incorporating a variety of these protein sources into the diet can ensure an adequate supply of essential amino acids necessary for managing autoimmune encephalitis and promoting overall brain health.

Carbohydrates and Fibers: Carbohydrates are the primary source of energy for the brain and body, making them essential for individuals with autoimmune encephalitis to maintain optimal cognitive function and overall health. However, not all carbohydrates are created equal, and consuming complex carbohydrates with a high fiber content is particularly beneficial. Complex carbohydrates provide a steady release of glucose into the bloodstream, preventing spikes and cr.

Healthy Fats and Omega-3s: Healthy fats, including monounsaturated and polyunsaturated fats, are essential for managing autoimmune encephalitis due to their anti-inflammatory properties and their role in maintaining the integrity of cell membranes in the brain.

Omega-3 fatty acids, in particular, have been extensively studied for their beneficial effects on neurological health and immune function. These essential fatty acids are integral components of neuronal membranes and are involved in modulating neurotransmitter signaling, synaptic plasticity, and neuroinflammation. Incorporating sources of omega-3s such as fatty fish (e.g., salmon, mackerel, sardines), flaxseeds, chia seeds, walnuts, and hemp seeds into the diet can help reduce inflammation and support cognitive function in individuals with autoimmune encephalitis. Additionally, replacing unhealthy trans fats and saturated fats with healthier alternatives like olive oil, avocado, and nuts can further promote brain health and overall well-being.

Vitamins and Minerals: Vitamins and minerals play essential roles in supporting immune function, neurotransmitter synthesis, antioxidant defense, and cellular energy production, all of which are crucial for managing autoimmune encephalitis and promoting neurological recovery. Deficiencies in certain vitamins and minerals, such as vitamin D, vitamin B12, folate, magnesium, and zinc, have been implicated in autoimmune diseases and neurological disorders, including encephalitis.

Therefore, ensuring adequate intake of these micronutrients through a balanced diet and, if necessary, supplementation is vital for optimizing immune function and neurological health. Foods rich in vitamins and minerals include leafy green vegetables, citrus fruits, berries, nuts, seeds, whole grains, lean meats, dairy products, and seafood.

By incorporating a diverse array of nutrient-dense foods into the diet, individuals with autoimmune encephalitis can support their body's natural healing processes and enhance overall resilience against inflammatory insults.

Antioxidants and Phytonutrients: Antioxidants and phytonutrients are powerful compounds found in plant-based foods that help neutralize harmful free radicals and reduce oxidative stress, thereby protecting against neuronal damage and inflammation in autoimmune encephalitis. These bioactive compounds have been shown to possess anti-inflammatory, neuroprotective, and immunomodulatory properties, making them valuable components of a therapeutic diet for managing autoimmune conditions. Fruits, vegetables, herbs, spices, teas, and nuts are abundant sources of antioxidants and phytonutrients, including flavonoids, polyphenols, carotenoids, and sulfur compounds. Consuming a diverse range of colorful plant foods can provide a spectrum of these beneficial compounds, each with its unique health-promoting properties. Moreover, incorporating herbs and spices such as turmeric, ginger, garlic, and cinnamon into meals can further enhance antioxidant intake and amplify the anti-inflammatory effects of the diet.

By harnessing the power of antioxidants and phytonutrients through dietary strategies, individuals with autoimmune encephalitis can support brain health, reduce inflammation, and promote overall well-being and resilience in the face of autoimmune challenges.

CHAPTER 4
CREATING A NUTRIENT-RICH DIET PLAN

Building Blocks of a Balanced Diet: A nutrient-rich diet plan is crucial for individuals managing autoimmune encephalitis, as it supports overall health and helps alleviate symptoms. The foundation of such a diet lies in understanding the building blocks of a balanced diet. This entails incorporating a variety of nutrients essential for brain function and immune system regulation. Key nutrients include carbohydrates, proteins, fats, vitamins, minerals, and water. Carbohydrates provide energy for the brain and body, and opting for complex carbohydrates such as whole grains, fruits, and vegetables ensures sustained energy release and stable blood sugar levels.

Proteins are vital for tissue repair and immune function, with sources like lean meats, fish, eggs, legumes, and dairy products being excellent choices. Healthy fats, found in sources like avocados, nuts, seeds, and fatty fish, are essential for brain health and reducing inflammation. Additionally, incorporating a wide range of vitamins and minerals through colorful fruits and vegetables supports immune function and overall well-being. Finally, staying hydrated is critical for cognitive function and detoxification processes within the body. By understanding these fundamental components of a balanced diet, individuals with autoimmune encephalitis can lay the groundwork for optimal nutrition to support their health journey.

Meal Planning Strategies: Effective meal planning is essential for ensuring consistency and adherence to a nutrient-rich diet plan for individuals with autoimmune encephalitis. One strategy involves establishing a routine for meals and snacks to maintain stable energy levels throughout the day. This includes consuming three balanced meals and incorporating nutritious snacks as needed to prevent energy dips and promote satiety. Furthermore, planning meals ahead of time allows for intentional ingredient selection and preparation methods to maximize nutrient retention and flavor. Meal prepping in batches can also save time and energy, making it easier to adhere to a healthy eating regimen, especially during busy periods. Another helpful strategy is to diversify food choices to ensure a wide range of nutrients and flavors, thereby preventing dietary monotony and enhancing satisfaction with meals. Additionally, involving family members or caregivers in meal planning and preparation can foster a supportive environment and promote adherence to dietary recommendations.

By implementing these meal planning strategies, individuals with autoimmune encephalitis can effectively manage their condition and support overall health and well-being.

 Foods to Include and Avoid: When creating a nutrient-rich diet plan for autoimmune encephalitis, it is essential to prioritize foods that support brain health, reduce inflammation, and boost immune function while minimizing or avoiding those that may exacerbate symptoms or trigger immune responses.

Foods to include in the diet are primarily whole, minimally processed foods rich in nutrients and antioxidants.

 This includes a variety of colorful fruits and vegetables, which provide essential vitamins, minerals, and phytonutrients with anti-inflammatory properties.

Incorporating sources of healthy fats such as avocados, olive oil, nuts, and seeds can help reduce inflammation and support cognitive function. Additionally, including lean proteins like fish, poultry, tofu, and legumes provides essential amino acids for tissue repair and immune support.

Whole grains like quinoa, brown rice, and oats are excellent sources of complex carbohydrates, fiber, and B vitamins, supporting sustained energy and gut health. On the other hand, certain foods should be limited or avoided, including highly processed foods, refined sugars, and trans fats, which can promote inflammation and impair immune function.

Individuals may also consider eliminating potential trigger foods such as gluten, dairy, and nightshade vegetables, as they may exacerbate autoimmune reactions in some individuals. By carefully selecting foods to include and avoid, individuals with autoimmune encephalitis can optimize their diet to support symptom management and overall well-being.

CHAPTER 5

SUPPORTING BRAIN HEALTH WITH DIET AND SUPPLEMENTS

Nutritional Strategies For Cognitive Function:

Nutritional strategies play a crucial role in supporting cognitive function, especially in individuals dealing with autoimmune encephalitis. Research suggests that certain nutrients can positively impact brain health and cognitive performance.

For instance, omega-3 fatty acids found in fish oil have been linked to improved cognitive function and may help reduce inflammation in the brain, which is particularly relevant in autoimmune conditions. Additionally, antioxidants such as vitamins C and E, as well as flavonoids found in fruits and vegetables, have been associated with cognitive benefits and may help protect brain cells from damage caused by oxidative stress. Moreover, adequate intake of B vitamins, particularly vitamin B12 and folate, is essential for maintaining healthy cognitive function as they play key roles in neurotransmitter synthesis and methylation processes.

Furthermore, incorporating foods rich in choline, such as eggs and lean meats, can support brain health by contributing to the production of acetylcholine, a neurotransmitter involved in memory and learning. Overall, adopting a well-rounded and nutrient-dense diet that includes a variety of fruits, vegetables, whole grains, lean proteins, and healthy fats can provide the essential nutrients needed to support cognitive function and overall brain health in individuals with autoimmune encephalitis.

Hydration is a fundamental aspect of overall health and well-being, and its importance is particularly heightened in individuals with autoimmune encephalitis. Proper hydration is essential for maintaining optimal brain function, as even mild dehydration can impair cognitive performance and exacerbate symptoms associated with autoimmune conditions affecting the brain. Dehydration can lead to decreased blood flow to the brain, resulting in reduced oxygen and nutrient delivery to brain cells, which may further exacerbate inflammation and oxidative stress. Moreover, dehydration can impair the body's ability to regulate temperature and remove toxins, potentially exacerbating symptoms and compromising overall health. Therefore, individuals with autoimmune encephalitis must prioritize adequate hydration by consuming an adequate amount of water and fluids throughout the day. Additionally, incorporating hydrating foods such as fruits and vegetables, which have high water content, can further support hydration levels. Monitoring hydration status and ensuring adequate fluid intake is essential for optimizing brain health and overall well-being in individuals with autoimmune encephalitis.

Additional Considerations:

Supplements can be valuable adjuncts to dietary strategies for supporting brain health in individuals with autoimmune encephalitis, but they should be used judiciously and under the guidance of healthcare professionals. Certain supplements have shown promise in supporting cognitive function and managing symptoms associated with autoimmune conditions affecting the brain. For example, omega-3 fatty acid supplements, particularly those rich in eicosapentaenoic acid (EPA) and docosahexaenoic acid (DHA), have been studied for their anti-inflammatory properties and potential benefits in reducing neuroinflammation and cognitive decline. Additionally, antioxidants such as vitamin E, vitamin C, and coenzyme Q10 may help protect brain cells from oxidative damage and support overall brain health. Furthermore, certain herbs and botanicals, such as turmeric and ginkgo biloba, have been studied for their potential neuroprotective effects and ability to modulate inflammatory pathways in the brain. However, it is important to note that supplement efficacy can vary depending on factors such as dosage, formulation, and individual response, and some supplements may interact with medications or exacerbate underlying health conditions.

Therefore, individuals with autoimmune encephalitis should consult with a healthcare professional before starting any new supplement regimen to ensure safety and efficacy. Additionally, supplements should be viewed as complementary to a healthy diet and lifestyle, rather than a substitute for nutrient-rich foods. Overall, supplement considerations should be individualized based on specific nutritional needs, underlying health conditions, and treatment goals in individuals with autoimmune encephalitis.

CHAPTER 6

LIFESTYLE FACTORS AND AUTOIMMUNE ENCEPHALITIS MANAGEMENT

To manage autoimmune encephalitis, which is characterized by brain inflammation caused by an autoimmune response, stress management techniques are crucial. Because chronic stress can aggravate autoimmune conditions by dysregulating the immune system and increasing inflammation, individuals with autoimmune encephalitis must implement effective stress management techniques.

Individuals with autoimmune encephalitis should prioritize establishing good sleep habits, which are essential for immune function, cognitive function, and overall health.

Poor sleep habits, such as irregular sleep schedules, exposure to electronic screens before bedtime, and late-day caffeine consumption, can disrupt the sleep-wake cycle and negatively impact immune function.

Exercise and movement are integral components of autoimmune encephalitis management. Regular physical activity has numerous benefits for overall health, including reducing inflammation, improving immune function, enhancing mood, and supporting cognitive function.

However, it's essential to approach exercise cautiously and adapt activities to individual capabilities and limitations, considering the potential neurological symptoms associated with autoimmune encephalitis.

Low-impact exercises such as walking, swimming, yoga, tai chi, or gentle stretching can be beneficial for improving mobility, flexibility, and strength without exacerbating symptoms.

Moreover, incorporating activities that promote balance, coordination, and proprioception can help address any neurological deficits and enhance overall functional capacity.

Individuals with autoimmune encephalitis must work closely with healthcare professionals, such as physical therapists or exercise physiologists, to develop personalized exercise programs tailored to their specific needs and goals.

 Additionally, listening to the body's cues, pacing oneself, and prioritizing rest and recovery are essential principles to uphold while engaging in physical activity to prevent overexertion and minimize the risk of symptom exacerbation.

Overall, adopting a holistic approach that integrates stress management techniques, healthy sleep habits, and appropriate exercise and movement recommendations is essential for optimizing outcomes and enhancing the quality of life for individuals living with autoimmune encephalitis.

CHAPTER 7
SPECIAL CONSIDERATIONS AND CHALLENGES

Dealing With Food Sensitivity And Allergy:

Individuals diagnosed with autoimmune encephalitis often face challenges related to food sensitivities and allergies. The immune system's dysregulation characteristic of autoimmune disorders can lead to heightened reactivity to certain foods, triggering adverse reactions. Identifying and managing these sensitivities is paramount for enhancing overall well-being and mitigating symptoms associated with the condition. A comprehensive approach involves conducting thorough assessments to pinpoint specific triggers, which may require collaboration between patients, healthcare professionals, and dietitians specializing in autoimmune disorders.

Elimination diets, where potential allergens are removed from the diet and systematically reintroduced, can be instrumental in identifying problematic foods. Additionally, incorporating anti-inflammatory foods and supplements known to support immune function, such as omega-3 fatty acids and probiotics, may help alleviate symptoms and reduce the risk of exacerbating food sensitivities. Furthermore, fostering an understanding of cross-reactivity between certain foods and environmental allergens is crucial in avoiding inadvertent exposure. Ultimately, personalized dietary plans tailored to individual needs and sensitivities can significantly contribute to managing autoimmune encephalitis and promoting overall health.

Addressing Medication Interactions:

Managing autoimmune encephalitis often involves the use of various medications aimed at modulating the immune response, reducing inflammation, and managing symptoms. However, individuals undergoing pharmacological treatment may encounter challenges related to medication interactions, which can impact treatment efficacy and overall health outcomes.

Healthcare providers need to conduct comprehensive evaluations of patients' medication regimens, considering potential interactions with dietary components and supplements. Certain foods and nutrients may interfere with the absorption, metabolism, or efficacy of medications commonly prescribed for autoimmune encephalitis, necessitating careful monitoring and adjustment of dietary intake. For instance, grapefruit and its derivatives contain compounds known to inhibit cytochrome P450 enzymes, which play a crucial role in drug metabolism, potentially leading to increased drug concentrations and adverse effects. Moreover, supplements such as St. John's Wort and garlic may induce or inhibit drug-metabolizing enzymes, altering medication levels in the body. Therefore, patients must communicate openly with their healthcare providers about their dietary habits and supplement use to minimize the risk of adverse interactions and optimize treatment outcomes.

Navigating The Social And Emotional Dimensions Of Dietary Changes:

The journey of managing autoimmune encephalitis extends beyond medical interventions to encompass various social and emotional dimensions, particularly concerning dietary changes. Adopting and adhering to dietary modifications can evoke a range of emotions, including frustration, anxiety, and social isolation, as individuals navigate unfamiliar dietary restrictions and limitations. It is imperative to recognize and address these psychosocial factors to support patients' overall well-being and adherence to dietary recommendations. Healthcare providers play a crucial role in offering empathy, guidance, and practical strategies to help patients cope with the emotional challenges associated with dietary changes. Encouraging open communication and providing resources for peer support groups or counseling services can empower individuals to express their concerns and seek assistance when needed. Moreover, fostering a supportive environment within familial and social circles can mitigate feelings of isolation and facilitate adherence to dietary modifications. Engaging in activities that promote self-care and stress management, such as mindfulness practices or hobbies, can also contribute to resilience and emotional well-being amidst dietary adjustments. By addressing the social and emotional aspects of dietary changes, healthcare providers can enhance patient satisfaction, treatment adherence, and overall quality of life for individuals managing autoimmune encephalitis.

CHAPTER 8
RECIPES AND MEAL IDEAS

Recipes and Meal Ideas for Individuals Managing Autoimmune Encephalitis play a crucial role in supporting their overall health and well-being. A balanced and nutrient-dense diet can help reduce inflammation, support the immune system, and promote brain health, all of which are essential in effectively managing autoimmune conditions. This section delves into various meal options, including breakfast, lunch, and dinner recipes, snack ideas, and desserts, tailored to

Breakfast Options: Breakfast is often considered the most important meal of the day, providing essential nutrients and energy to kickstart the day. For individuals with autoimmune encephalitis, it is critical to choose breakfast options that are rich in nutrients known to support brain health and reduce inflammation. Incorporating foods high in antioxidants, omega-3 fatty acids, vitamins, and minerals can help protect the brain from oxidative stress and inflammation.

Incorporating a variety of nutrient-dense foods into the diet during lunch and dinner is a great way to support overall health and well-being. Combining lean proteins, whole grains, healthy fats, and a colorful array of fruits and vegetables can provide the body with essential nutrients while also satisfying hunger and cravings. Grilled

Snack Ideas and Desserts: Individuals with autoimmune encephalitis can incorporate snacks and desserts into a balanced diet, provided they are made with nutritious ingredients and consumed in moderation. Choosing snacks that are high in protein, healthy fats, and fiber can help stabilize blood sugar levels and prevent energy crashes throughout the day. Some snack ideas may include Greek yogurt with berries and almonds, hummus with raw vegetables, or an apple slice.

recipes and meal ideas tailored to individuals with autoimmune encephalitis should focus on incorporating nutrient-dense foods that support brain health, reduce inflammation, and promote overall well-being. By choosing foods rich in antioxidants, omega-3 fatty acids, vitamins, and minerals, individuals can effectively manage their condition and improve their quality of life. Experimenting with various ingredients and recipes can help individuals find

CHAPTER 9
RESOURCES AND FURTHER SUPPORT

Recommended Reading & Websites:

A crucial aspect of managing autoimmune encephalitis (AE) is staying informed about the condition and its treatment options. There exists a plethora of literature and online resources dedicated to educating patients, caregivers, and healthcare professionals about AE. Recommended reading materials often include authoritative textbooks, scientific journals, and patient-friendly guides. Textbooks such as "Autoimmune Encephalitis" by Josep Dalmau and Francesc Graus provide in-depth insights into the pathophysiology, clinical manifestations, diagnosis, and management strategies of AE.

Scientific journals like Neurology, Lancet Neurology, and the Journal of Neuroimmunology regularly publish research articles and reviews pertinent to AE. For individuals seeking easily accessible and comprehensive information, reputable websites like the Autoimmune Encephalitis Alliance (AE Alliance), Encephalitis Society, and National Institute of Neurological Disorders and Stroke (NINDS) offer valuable resources, including fact sheets, webinars, and patient stories. These resources not only empower patients and caregivers with knowledge but also facilitate communication with healthcare providers, thereby promoting collaborative decision-making and better health outcomes.

Supporting Groups And Communities:

Living with AE can be challenging, both emotionally and physically, for patients and their loved ones.

Support groups and online communities play a vital role in providing encouragement, empathy, and practical advice to individuals affected by AE. These groups serve as safe spaces where patients and caregivers can share their experiences, express concerns, and seek guidance from others who understand their struggles firsthand. Platforms like Facebook, Reddit, and Inspire host numerous AE-specific groups where members engage in discussions on topics ranging from symptom management and treatment options to coping strategies and advocacy efforts. Additionally, organizations such as the AE Alliance and the Encephalitis Society often facilitate in-person support groups, webinars, and annual conferences, fostering connections among individuals affected by AE and fostering a sense of community. Through these supportive networks, patients and caregivers not only find emotional solace but also gain valuable insights into navigating the complexities of AE and accessing resources for holistic well-being.

Consulting With Health Care Professionals:

Effective management of AE necessitates a multidisciplinary approach involving various healthcare professionals, including neurologists, immunologists, psychiatrists, neuropsychologists, and dietitians. Consulting with knowledgeable and experienced healthcare providers is paramount for accurate diagnosis, personalized treatment planning, and ongoing monitoring of disease progression. Neurologists specializing in autoimmune diseases possess the expertise to conduct comprehensive neurological evaluations, order relevant diagnostic tests (e.g., MRI, EEG, CSF analysis), and prescribe appropriate immunotherapy (e.g., corticosteroids, IVIG, rituximab). Immunologists play a crucial role in assessing immune system dysregulation, conducting antibody testing, and exploring targeted immunomodulatory therapies. Psychiatrists and neuropsychologists contribute to the management of neuropsychiatric symptoms, cognitive deficits, and emotional well-being through psychotherapy, pharmacotherapy, and cognitive rehabilitation interventions. Furthermore, dietitians knowledgeable in neurology and autoimmune disorders can offer tailored nutritional guidance, including anti-inflammatory diets, supplementation recommendations, and strategies to address dysphagia and feeding difficulties. Collaborating with a coordinated team of healthcare professionals ensures comprehensive care, optimizes treatment outcomes, and enhances the overall quality of life for individuals living with AE.

CONCLUSION

In conclusion, nutrition plays a pivotal role in the management and rehabilitation of autoimmune encephalitis (AE), a complex neurological disorder characterized by immune-mediated inflammation of the brain.

Adopting a holistic approach to nutrition that encompasses understanding, nutrient essentials, meal planning, brain health strategies, lifestyle tips, special considerations, and delicious recipes is essential for enhancing well-being and resilience in individuals affected by AE.

By optimizing nutrient intake, supporting immune function, reducing inflammation, and promoting neuroplasticity, a well-balanced diet tailored to individual needs can complement medical interventions and contribute to improved clinical outcomes and quality of life.

However, navigating nutritional challenges associated with AE, such as dysphagia, dysphonia, dysphoria, dysautonomia, and dietary restrictions, requires careful consideration, multidisciplinary collaboration, and ongoing support from healthcare professionals, caregivers, and support networks.

Furthermore, continued research, education, and advocacy efforts are needed to raise awareness, address knowledge gaps, and promote access to evidence-based nutrition interventions for individuals living with AE.

By embracing the principles of nutrition therapy and fostering a supportive ecosystem of care, we can empower patients and caregivers to navigate the journey of AE with resilience, hope, and dignity.